D1585788

Easy Aromatherapy Recipes For Beginners

An everyday guide to using simple, organic and affordable essential oils at home

Fiona Summers

Introduction

Welcome to the magical world of aromatherapy. Its wonderful scents typify luxury and it is a delicious way to pamper yourself and those you love.

Did you know though, that the essential oils have really potent healing effects too?

In this book I will take you step by step how to choose the right oils for different conditions. There are recipes to help you blend mixes to put a spring in your step and a song in your heart.

Not only that, I will walk you hand in hand along the shop counter and explain how to choose your first few bottles and what to look for to check you are paying a good price.

Within days you could have your home transformed into a loving and harmonious environment and be feeling blissfully relaxed and calm. Without making many changes at all your family will be happier and calmer. You will learn how to get the kids through exams with better grades and far less effort, just by using essential oils. We can even put some sensuality into your relationship too.

Whoever said you will never find the answer to your problems at the bottom of a bottle had never read this book! A bottle of essential oils can ease away the pain of an aching back and an aching heart too. Used right in the right way they can make your spirit completely soar.

So without further ado…turn the page and let me lead you into the wonderland that is aromatherapy.

Disclaimer

Terms of Use: This book has been written by a professionally qualified and practicing aromatherapist. Although the author and publisher have made every effort to ensure that the information in this book is accurate and complete, they do not warrant the accuracy of the information, text and graphics contained within the book due to the rapidly changing nature of science, research, known and unknown facts and internet. The Author and the publisher do not hold any responsibility for errors, omissions or contrary interpretation of the subject matter herein. This book is presented solely for motivational and informational purposes only.

For further details please see the detailed safety information and full disclaimer at the end of the book before going any further.

How to use this book

The book is designed to be used in three separate parts. The first gives you a little background on how the plant matter used by as far back as the Ancient Egyptians has become the massive growth market it is today. It explains how the concentrated essences are drawn from the plants and how you can use them to bring about health.

In section two we look at some of the most important oils and how you can use them in your everyday life to bring about healing. This quick reference guide will enable you to see at a glance how effectively you will be able to use and oil and whether it will give you good value for money.

The final section is a breakdown of some of my favourite essential oil recipes. Tried and tested concoctions which will have you feeling wonderful and looking great.

I hope you enjoy exploring the world of aromatherapy as much as I do. Very quickly you discover that there is much more to being well than meets the eye. Often it is as much today with how you feel in your heart about life which translates into vibrant and happy healthiness. Essential oils help you to capture that sparkle in the eye.

So what are you waiting for?

Let's dive right in!

Contents

What is aromatherapy?

Aromatherapy is the use of concentrated essences of plants to bring about wellness. We call these essences essential oils. They can be extracted from leaves, barks, grasses and flower petals. Each and every one of them has their own special healing abilities.

In its truest form aromatherapy is an extremely profound healing skill. A professional aromatherapist is not only an expert in the effects each oil will have but many other aspects of health too. Aromatherapy works on the principle that for a person to feel well, they must be balanced in their mind, their body and their spiritual life too. Essential oils are extremely helpful in bringing about these changes.

As a therapy, it falls under the title of complementary medicine; that is, it is meant to work alongside the traditional medicines which the doctor gives you. It is important never to replace your prescribed medicine with essential oils without consent from your general practitioner. In most cases though, the two treatments work on entirely different body systems and will sit happily together, there are a couple of provisos though.

Essential oils affect blood sugar and the way the body manufactures insulin and so patients with diabetes should avoid some aromatherapy recipes. The same applies for suffers of epilepsy and pregnant women too. This is covered in more detail here.

Aromatherapy? Where did it even come from?

The History of Aromatherapy

To find the beginnings of this complementary medicine we must travel back in time to way before the birth of Christ. We have to run top speed past the lions and the ferocious gladiators in the Coliseums, back through the ages of the Cyclops and the myths of the Ancient Greeks, to the first building blocks being placed at the foot of the pyramids.

The earliest usage of oils which we can definitively date is to the ancient Egyptians who were fierce ambassadors of their usage. Indeed much of what we know about the oils is built on the learning we gained from them.

Archaeological digs have uncovered ancient tears of frankincense and myrrh in tombs, which we know played a large part not only in their embalming processes but also in the way connected with their gods and goddesses in prayer.

You are likely to recognise these from a certain famous story in the bible which dates back just over 2000 years. When the magi brought these gifts for the Christ-Child the precious resins they bought were far more financially valuable then gold, and also gave prediction that He would die as a king. At that time Myrrh was the embalming oil reserved only for Pharoahs.

Through the ages Myrrh has been used extensively by ancient doctors because of its skin healing qualities, but also its abilities to guard against infection. Roman soldiers would all proceed onto the battlefield with a pouch of the tree sap on their belts. We know this from some ancient writings by a man called Galen. He was a doctor to the Roman armies and he is often referred to as the father of medicine.

Galen used plants for healing extensively but he was the first of the medical profession to understand the development of disease. During these times people believed that afflictions were fated; that any illness had been sent by the some kind of supernatural force. He is recorded as telling his peers that is was important to watch, and to observe any developments of an illness. We live in a world where diagnosis was the norm, but this investigation of the prognosis of disease was revolutionary.

Pliny the Elder was a naturalist who wrote extensively about the healing effects of the plant world. His beautiful work the Materia Medica is full of extremely detailed drawings. This was the only one of his works which survived his death in the eruption of Pompeii. For this we have a very definitive date of AD79.

Strangely right across the other side of the world (which of course was then flat!) the Arabs were using plants for healing too, but in an entirely different manner. Still plant medicine, but we can see in the writings of Avicenna (you can also search him under the name of Ali Abu Ibn Cinna) they were *distilling* plant essences. These distilled essences are the very things which we refer to as essential oils.

Hmm, twentieth first century buzzword…..could there be more to this, I wonder?

Let's travel forward a bit then. We'll skip to the 16th century since there is little evidence to show you from the Dark Ages.

By the 16th century though, most large houses across Europe had their own still houses. They made digestive concoctions from herbs but also floral essences from lavender, roses and the like. They had long perfected capturing the qualities of their native plants but as the crusaders came back from the East, they bought with them such treasures as the Western world had never seen before. Suddenly the potential for blending was boundless.

As the Age of Reason dawned in the 18th and 19th Centuries medicine changed. Doctors understood diseases as we know them, but they were also beginning understand how to dissect the oils, isolate active ingredients and synthesize them.

This will be explained in more detail but imagine if you can, the streets of London teaming with addicts struggling with their addiction to Laudanum. The precursor to heroin, this derivative of the opium poppy was the epidemic sweeping the world. No wonder plants began to go out of favour.

Plant medicine, now cast out as medieval superstition belonging to quacks, still managed to garner the interest of the fascinated few. In 1926 a paper by a Frenchman called Renée Gattefosse refers to a shocking discovery that plant essences are working more effectively than the synthetic antiseptics he is using in the hospital. The sweet smelling essences proved him to coin the term "aromatherapie", which is from where the term is derived.

Mutterings and stirrings were carried across the medical world on the breeze and throughout the 20s and 30s naturopathy began to gain momentum. Papers were written and experiments were done in a flourish of excitement to find if the word on the street were true. Somehow though, they could not break through the core of the medical world. That is, until Dr Jean Valnet burned his hand…and then aromatherapy was changed for ever

Valnet had been working in his lab and suffered an agonizing burn. Looking for the closes thing to cool his hand he plunged it into a vat of lavender oil (which always strikes me as incredibly lucky, what if it had been sulphuric acid?) instantly the pain began to subside.

Over the days to come, he watches in astonishment as the tissues of the burn began to remedy and heal themselves far quicker than he could ever have expected. Free from scarring, he resolved to spend the rest of his life advertising the benefits of plants in healing. This he did, until his death in 1995.

In the sixties aromatherapy developed in a very radically different way. Whilst previously scholars had concentrated on the physical healing effects of the plant essences, now flower children began to experiment with plants as hallucinogenics. Smoking all manner of goodness-knows-what, the sparks of understanding between the connections of the mind-body-spirit principles were formed. For the first time we started to understand how plants could affect our emotions and open our minds to truths which perhaps in normal day to day activities we may not be able to hear.

So with popularity and just a sprinkle of knowledge here and a dust of expertise here, it became important to legislate and monitor aromatherapy. Governing and official bodies were formed with their own sets of examinations. Essential oil therapy now links arms with reflexology, acupressure, chiropractic and counselling skills as well as vitamin therapy, massage and diet to create the very thorough and deeply penetrating approach to wellness it is today.

How Are Essential Oils Made?

It stands to reason some plants will give up their juices more easily than others. Lemon oil for instance is far easier to gather than an essential oil from cinnamon bark, so a variety of different methods are used to collect the essences. Almost all rely on the basic principle that oil and water do not mix.

Fractional Distillation

This is the most extensively used method of extraction. The purists of aromatherapy would tell you that only oils which have been extracted by this matter can truly be called essential oils, but that is not a commonly held belief.

Plant matter is collected together in a vat and then high pressure steam is purged through it. The steam goes up a tube and then as it cools the water collects in another vat. The oil which has been drawn from the plant sits on the top.

In fact there are two separate products here: the essential oil and the water which also has very minute traces of the oil in. It has the fragrance of the plant and also has its very dilute properties. We call these floral waters or hydrolats. You may have come across rosewater which is an example of these.

Cohabition

The most important aspect of aromatherapy is it is imperative the whole plant must be used. In certain types of fractional distillation some parts of the chemical constituents are left behind. Rose otto for instance loses its phenyl ethyl alcohol in the process. This is the part of the oil which gives the oil its fragrance.

In cohabition this alcohol is distilled again and then added back to the rest of the oil.

Enfleurage

This is a very costly method and is no longer widely used for commercial production. It has been performed the same way for centuries.

Trays are smeared with vegetable fat and are covered with thousands of petals. The most common of these are rose petals. These are then laid out in the hot sun. The vegetable fat absorbs the essential oils from the petals. The petals are then replaced with fresh ones.

This is performed over and over until the fat is entirely saturated with oil. Then the fat mixture is then washed with alcohol for only a very pure essential oil is left behind. This method makes an incredibly high quality product.

Expression

This is a relatively cheap process mainly used for citrus fruits. Essential oils are drawn from the peels of the fruits. A method called Écuelle a piqué runs very sharp needles through the rind and then it is pressed hard to release the oils from the rind. There are some bi-products of this process, water etc contaminate it so then it is put into a centrifuge to separate these off from the pure oil.

It is important to remember that this method (also called cold pressing) has no steps to clean the oil. The rind can be subject to a great deal of pesticide spraying in intensive farming. Therefore the oils made through this method can have very large concentrations of the chemicals.

Solvent Extraction

We talked earlier about frankincense and myrrh. These are resins which are notoriously unhelpful in giving up their essences and so these have to be dissolved by solvents. We call these solvents concretes.

Dependant on which concrete is used there is usually a residue of left behind. For this reason often these can be dismissed as inferior quality essential oils. Historically benzene would be used which can leave behind as much as 20% residue but now it is recognised as having carcinogenic risks and so hexane has pretty much replaced it. This leaves around 6-10% residue.

The most effective concrete is CO_2 Extraction which leaves behind no residue. Carbon dioxide of CO_2 becomes hypercritical at 33 degrees Fahrenheit. What this means is at this point it is neither liquid nor gas. By placing the plant matter into a high pressure chamber at this point the CO_2 collects the essential oil. Then all that needs to happen is the pressure needs to be removed and the CO_2 simply disappears into the air leaving behind an extremely pure oil.

Maceration

Whist not strictly speaking essential oils, I have added this in because it makes a lovely way to start experimenting. In macerations you take some plant matter and leave them to soak in a carrier oil. The simplest ones make lovely salad oils like rosemary in olive oil, but you can develop it to catch the properties of your most favourite flowers too.

How to use essential oils

In order to work their magic essential oils need to be absorbed into the body. There are two main ways to do this.

I.   Inhalation
II. Through the skin

Inhalation

In some ways the term aromatherapy is a misnomer, as it implies it is the scent of the oils which make them effective. This is not correct. The oils are complex blends of many chemical constituents, each of these create different actions in the body. When we breathe in the oils they travel up the nose via the sinuses, pass through the olfactory system and limbic systems and flush around the brain affecting not only emotions but also releasing hormones too.

The limbic system of our brain is responsible for how we learn, our memories and our emotions. I suppose this is what we would term as our minds.

The sinuses are unusual in that they are the only nerves which travel directly to the brain. All others travel along the spinal cord inside of the spinal column, which means that when oils are inhaled changes in the body will happen very quickly.

This is a wonderful way to affect emotions, to get a quick happy shot or a chill pill, but also it's great for un-bunging stopped up noses too.

Through the skin

You may see this also described as "trans-dermally", which is the clever kids' version for saying the same thing!

The skin is the largest organ in the body, it also is semi-permeable. The molecules in essential oils are small enough to absorb through the pores of the skin and into the circulatory system. There they flush around the blood stream and go to the parts of the body which need them. These trigger the brain to produce the hormones which balance the body's internal workings and help to bring about healing.

Often when I first started in aromatherapy, twenty years ago, people used to look at me in disbelief and say "so if I rub this cream on my forehead it will cure my headache?" which always seemed a bit odd that they would more readily accept that swallowing a pill might do better. 5 minutes after they had applied the oils you could see their conversion to alternative therapies happening before your very eyes!

In total, it takes around 20 minutes for the skin to fulfil its action of osmosis and for the oils to be fully absorbed.

It is important to remember these oils are *concentrated* essences of plants. They are extremely potent and in some cases will burn the skin. Therefore it is important you always dilute essential oils in some kind of carrier before use.

Carriers

Carrier oils

The most simplistic of carriers is a standard vegetable oil. There are some beautiful ones on the market all of which have their own wonderfully healing qualities which will enhance essential oils blends. All you need for dilution purposes though is some basic cooking oil, sunflower, grapeseed, or olive perhaps. These make wonderful starting points for massage.

Dilution is so small you will wonder whether you have read my notes right, but in 4 fl oz of oil you need no more than 10 drops of essential oils. You can find out more about dilution here.

More Exotic Carrier Oils

Carrier oils are usually macerations of plants so they do not have the potency essential oils do, but they change the textures and feels of your products as well as enhancing their healing properties. Be aware that many carrier oils are made from the kernels of fruits and also from nuts. Any of these would therefore not be suitable for use if you suffer from a nut allergy.

When you tire of using the sunflower, olive or groundnut oils you have in your pantry, here are some more you may enjoy experimenting with:

Evening Primrose - A thick, rich, gloopy bright yellow oil which is full of GLA which is wonderfully healing to the skin. Perfect for eczema and psoriasis but also for gynaecological care too.

Borage – This is a lovely light, fairly colourless oil. It has connections to the liver and so is very helpful in treating any condition which could be exacerbated by stress.

St John's Wort – Bright red, a beautiful berry of an oil. It is very healing for aches and pains, but also is helpful with treating symptoms of stress incontinence. You must however check with your doctor before using this oil as St Johns Worth can neutralise the effects of a handful of prescription drugs. Get your doctor to check this for you.

Jasmin – A rich, heady thick and luscious golden yellow oil. It is wonderful for skin care and also very helpful in treating conditions with scarring.

Calendula – A cheaper alternative to the essential oil this is a very caring skin healer.

Hazelnut (*Nut) – The very best oil I have found for exfoliating the skin. Perfect for mixing into scrubs of facial massage treatments.

In The Bath

Putting essential oils in the bath is one of the most effective ways to use them. Remember the skin being an organ, visualize how each pore in the body opens in the warmth of the water and allows the oil access to the body. The warmth softens the muscles and it encourages the capillaries in the skin to move closer to the surface and welcome the oils.

At the same time the steam releases the molecules of the oils into the atmosphere so we can breathe them more easily too, relaxing us and helping us to switch off.

There is only one word we can say really here, isn't there.....aaaaahhhh!

For the full benefit of the aromatherapy bath, lie there for at least 20 minutes.

It is lovely to make bath gifts for birthdays and Christmas but actually there is such a large volume of water in a bath, there is no need for extra carriers. You should use no more than a total of 5 -10 drops into a bath of warm water.

Creams and Lotions

These are very under used, but to my mind they are the single most useful way to carry essential oils. They make great ways to be able to apply small amounts of oils little and often. They protect the skin from the potent oils and they are easy to make and use.

You can in effect use any plain cream and stir in some oils, but it is possible to buy blanks from beauty wholesalers and also some pharmacists. For those of you wish to experiment more I have included a recipe to make your own lotions.

Burners

These are also sometimes called evaporators or diffusers. Some run on electricity, others rely on a candle underneath a bowl of warmed water to release essential oils into the atmosphere. These work really well for changing the atmosphere of a room or for emanating scents which will deter insects, for instance.

Neat

There is always an exception to prove the rule. In this case there are two oils which you can, and in some cases should, use neat (that is undiluted) on the skin. These are lavender and tea tree which you may also see named as Maleleuca.

Lavender – Lavendula angustifolia

Think back to the notes on history and you may recall Dr Jean Valnet treating is burns with lavender oil. To this day we have not found a better burns treatment and neither would be need to search, neat lavender sprinkled liberally on burns and scalds is an amazing medicine. Put the injured area under a cold running tap for two minutes then pour lavender oil all over it.

As a teenager, I had beautiful skin when everyone else was covered in oozing pustular spots, because I knew the secret of lavender oil. I practically walked around with it glued to my chin. Neat lavender oil zaps zits…

Neat lavender on your temples can also relieve stress and ease tension headaches. Only use what comes on your finger when you touch the bottle though, as the scent can become nauseating.

Tea Tree – Maleleuca alternifolia

The properties of tea tree are anti-viral and antiseptic (amongst many others). It is the best first line of defence against bugs and infections. Look at the inside of your wrist and you will see a number of blue lines where the veins are close to the surface. Smear neat tea tree onto the wrist at the first sign of a sniffle or any indication that an infection may be threatened. Repeat every 20 minutes for 4 hours and the drop down to three times daily.

Lemon Oil- But only for warts!!! Be careful….

Lemon oil is extremely astringent and is a dermal irritant which means it will irritate your skin a great deal. It will however kill warts and verrucae if you dab it neat carefully onto the affected area with a cotton bud. Be very careful not to get the lemon oil onto the surrounding skin. Repeat daily.

Do not take internally

Many essential oils have extremely irritant qualities, not just to the skin but to mucous membranes too. Under no circumstances should you ingest essential oils. If it does happen accidentally, drink a pint of milk and visit the accident and emergency department of the hospital. Ensure you take the bottle with you so they can assess the dangers you may face from the offending plant.

Some illnesses do not react well to essential oils, for example: diabetes, epilepsy, pregnancy, and breast feeding mothers, For further information click here.

Dilution and Blending

It never ceases to amaze me how many drops of oil people put into a blend. Always employ the philosophy that less is more. This is for two reasons.

I.   Essential oils are expensive!
II. The oils are so potent. The body takes what it needs and then releases any surplus into the blood stream as waste. It brings a whole new dimension to throwing money down the toilet!

The very maximum you want to work to is a dilution of 1:25. That is to say for every 25 drops of carrier oil or base you will only want to add 1 drop of essential oil. I work to far less.

Usually one drop of an oil is effective in a blend, two if I want a sledgehammer approach and three drops in emergency situations.

At all times remember you can add more in the next treatment if you need to…but if you get it wrong and add to much you could burn yourself, end up fitting, affect your blood sugar or even your heart. Act sensibly and aromatherapy is your friend, be a fool and I promise you will know about it!!!!

Buying essential oils

It seems proper at this point to explain my comment earlier that essential oils are expensive. It is true, but there are good reasons for it. There are many factors which affect their prices.

These are:

I. Method of extraction – CO_2 costs far more than expression

II. Yield – some plants only generate small amounts of oil so far more plant matter is required.

III. Availability of plant matter – Some plants are seasonal or only grow in certain places

IV. Sustainable resources- Oils such as sandalwood have to be gained from specially grown trees.

V. Dilution – Some oils are what are called "cut" with other oils to make them easier for people to afford to buy. A good example of this is Lemon Balm oil or Melissa officianalis. Melissa (True) is 100% pure, Melissa (Type) has been cut with Lemon Verbena oil because Lemon balm leaves are notoriously hard to get much oil from.

All of these dictate how much an oil will cost you. Essential oil production is a huge economy but actually oil retailing prices do not vary that much, it is not particularly competitive. It is fair to say if a price seems lower than any others you have seen…there is probably a reason to think it may be of inferior quality.

Labelling should give you some pointers. Always check that the oil is shown with its English name but also its Latin name too. You should see it shown as *Lavendula latifolia.* Note how the first word is shown with a capital letter and the second is in small case? If a label differs from this there may be cause for concern. This method of labelling (called binomial nomenclature) will tell you which species of the family of plants an oil has been taken from. Certain chemotypes of an oil should be avoided.

In some parts of the world and especially on some MLM marketing websites, you may also see essential oils graded. You may see them denoted as *Grade A* or *therapeutic grade* oils. This is purely a marketing ploy; no such official legislation has ever been introduced.

The French, who are some of the planet's most prolific oil producers, have some governance from an organisation called AFNOR. This can be used as a guide to show you quality of the oil but not necessarily for therapeutic reasons. Afnor is solely concerned with the quality of the oil for the economic growth of the areas for export.

Your label will often show country of origin and this can be useful. Some areas of production naturally have less pollution and so are more pure. An Alpine lavender plant will be grown at such altitude it is way above the rigours of pollution. There are fewer of these plants and so this comes at a high price tag.

By contrast think of the scary things which pour into the soil and the air in war zones…oils taken from these areas tend to have sharpness to them from the pollution they have absorbed.

Look for organic oils for this reason; they are purer and more effective. As discussed before, if a label says CO2 extracted you have found a rather beautiful thing. You should give your purse a good shake and see if you can find a few extra pennies to spend on it.

Storing Essential Oils

When we start all of us make the same mistake. In fact, remember I have said this as you clear up your first mess! Essential oils degrade plastic. If you store a blend in a plastic bottle, sooner or later it is going to melt into a revolting greasy mess in your cupboard!

Store all essential oils products in dark glass bottles in a dark place.

Just like all organisms, plant essences are subject to oxidation. Over time the cells begin to die off and the oils lose their efficacy. Some oils oxidise faster than others. Citrus oils for instance begin to degrade after just 6 months. On the other hand I have a bottle of myrrh oil which is still going strong 15 years after I got it….it works but it's not got superman strength any longer.

Sunlight is like kryptonite to oils. It oxidises them far faster than anything else. Keep them dark and keep them cool.

When you do undo the top to use the oils, be aware that they are volatile and so molecules are escaping even if you are not pouring drops. Ensure you put the lid back on tight enough to stop the escape further.

Ensure you wash your hands after use (think about forgetting to wash chilli off your fingers and then rubbing your eyes but ten times as bad!) In fac,t I think my experience with rushing to the loo with citronella oil on my hands may have been even worse than that! Lordie….my eyes did run!!!!

Lastly, keep essential oils out of reach of children. Every one of my kids has loved having "Magic Eels" in the bath, and then thought about doing themselves when I've not been looking. The wrong oil in the bath can do just as much damage as scalding water. Worse too, some oils smell like sweeties. Remember Parma Violets? Violet oil smells exactly the same. Leaving essential oils around when there are curious fingers is a recipe for disaster.

What Are The Most Popular Oils Used For?

There are so many essential oils on the market you would have to collect for an entire lifetime before you completed the set. Then, the day after they buried you I can guarantee more would appear on the shelves. It's useful then to look at which ones make the most efficient ones. If you stock your box with one of each of the following you have the beginnings of a really good assortment to treat with.

Lavender – Lavendula officinalis

Everyone's favourite essential oil, it can be used for so many different things you could be forgiven for thinking aromatherapists use it as a cure all. We don't use it for everything, but yes….a lot of things certainly!

It is soothing and relaxing. They seem like two similar words but I use soothing as a physical response to pain, and relaxing in terms of emotionally. It will soothe the sting or itching out of skin disorders and it eases aches and pains. At the end of the day a few drops of lavender helps us to switch off and unwind ready for a lovely night's sleep.

It is such a gentle and benign oil, it is safe to use on the most vulnerable and delicate people. Babies are calmed and elderly people feel a relief from their rheumatic symptoms with lavender too.

We have spoken of burns and spots already, and how we would use lavender neat for these. Use it also in skin creams to balance the sebum in greasy teenage complexions.

Be careful of the lavender labelling as there are many chemotypes of this plant. Some are more "friendly" than others. Stick to Lavendula officinalis & angustifolia as your treatment bottles of choice.

Tea Tree Oil – Maleleuca alternifolia

What a wonderful oil this is! It is antiviral, anti-fungal, antibiotic, antiseptic…in short if there is a nasty you want rid of, pour some tea tree on it. I have seen it do amazing things with scratches that are infected. It is wonderful for cleaning down surfaces when there are bugs around. For sore throats, open the top of the bottle and gasp in the fumes. I also like to put a couple of drops in warm water and gargle to get rid of the soreness. It makes a wonderful astringent toner for greasy skin.

In this day and age of always wearing trainers and sneakers the incidence of athlete's foot seems to be on the rise. Pour it neat into the offending parts then also put a couple of drops in the final rinse in the washing machine to cleanse resides from socks too.

Geranium – Pelargonium graveolens

The cynical would call this poor man's rose oil since it will do the same job as its counterpart which costs at least ten times more. I, however think it is an incredibly magical oil in its own right.

For gynaecological complaints it is unsurpassed. Period pains, premenstrual tension, menstrual migraines and also the depression and mood swings which accompany menopausal changes all get incredible help from this sweet smelling oil.

It nourishes dry skin beautifully. Most of all, geranium oil *attacks* anxiety. A couple of drops in the bath at the end of the day and you can feel your worries simply drifting away from you. It really is a wonderful oil.

Chamomile Maroc - Ormenis multicaulis

There are three different types of Chamomile you can buy. All are spectacular healers but this one has the most uses and is usually the cheapest to buy of the three.

It is relaxing and soothing. I always use it for taking itching away from the skin. It is so incredibly sedative so if you have been very upset for a reason Camomile can very much work like an off switch.

It is ant-inflammatory (although its brother Roman Camomile *Anthemis nobilis* is more so) it will reduce swelling and also help to bring down bruising.

It is beautifully digestive, it will help everything from the griping pains of colic through the easing the cramps of diarrhoea. You may recognise its name from chamomile tea. It also has anti-spasmodic qualities which can be helpful in everything from relief from ongoing coughing through the cramp in the lags.

This is a most versatile oil. I feel it is a bit of a supporting act though rather than the star of the show. Mix it with other oils to increase their healing powers.

Peppermint – Mentha piperita

The bright iciness of the mint plant will put a zing in anyone's step, but it hides a rather machiavellian secret. For peppermint will render any homeopathic remedies completely useless. Never take peppermint in any form if you are also receiving treatments from a homeopath.

That aside, this refreshing oil can bring about some lovely effects. It is deliciously refreshing, so it really works well to add into invigorating mixes like shower gels. One drop in a bowl of water will make you feel like you have traded in your feet for a new pair. It also is glorious in foot rubs and creams too for the same reason.

It is digestive (which is one of the reasons we have lamb with mint sauce) it breaks down fats and provokes the digestive enzymes. Make it your first port of call if you have heartburn or digestion.

Peppermint is a tonic for the liver, and is excellent for helping to ease the effects of stress. Use this oil with care though as it is a very wakeful plant....put it in your bath in the evening and you will still be tossing and turning at 3am.

This is an oil best avoided in pregnancy.

Eucalyptus – Eucalyptus globulus
This will be a familiar scent to you. It has a clinical smell which is reminiscent of having a cold. That is because most cold and flu preparations have a splash of this oil in. It is the most wonderfully powerful decongestant. It can cut through catarrh quickly and efficiently.

It is also a tonic for the liver and is helpful for reducing stress headaches.

Myrrh – Commiphora myrrha
This bitter smelling and frustratingly slow-to-get-out-of-the-bottle oil is an amazing skin healer. Add to ointments to clean cracks and cuts and help them to heal over far more quickly.

It is decongestant too, so it is great if you have a cold.

Myrrh is a great oil to choose if you suffer from premenstrual syndrome. It acts as a tonic to the womb, strengthening it and helping to reduce clotting and therefore pain. For the same reason it is often used to help ladies who are in established labour. It is important not to use it though, until labour has been confirmed.

You may want to check safety data for pregnancy.

Rosemary – Rosemarinus officinalis
Another one of these traditional culinary herbs, rosemary is excellent for helping digest fatty foods (another roast lamb partner, did you notice?)

Rosemary has two extraordinary qualities: the first is how effectively it will help nerve pain; that can be sciatica, tooth ache, neuralgia anything where a nerve is inflamed. The second is it will increase blood flow and circulation to the surface of the skin. For this reason it is undergoing a great deal of research into it possible benefits in the fight against hair loss.

Used in a sensible health regime and diet, it can help to reduce cholesterol.

It is an extraordinary oil but it does have safety concerns for epilepsy sufferers.

Lemon Balm Oil – Melissa officinalis
There are two types of this oil (Type and True). Melissa Type is every bit as efficacious as True and so do not fear you are buying an inferior product. It is not, it is simply not as strong.

Melissa oil has the most incredible effects on suffers of dementia. It helps them to connect with their environment and when blended with lavender oil is recommended by health professionals to help reduce challenging behaviour and distress.

A natural antihistamine it is a magnificent help for reducing effects of allergies. This is very helpful in the summer hay fever season but it can be every bit as effective for cat/ dog allergies etc.

I call it liquid sunshine. It lifts your spirits and always induces a smile. It is particularly helpful if someone is exhausted from long term stress as it can help to rebuild resilience.

Marigold – Calendula officinalis or Tagetes glandulifera
I have included both marigolds here as they are very different but both entirely wondrous. Marigold is THE best skin healer you will ever find. For generations we have been relying on it to protect our precious babies' bums from nappy rash but now excitingly science has found an even more important use for it.

Calendula (which is the pot marigold you have in the garden) is now recommended to breast cancer patients after they have had radiation therapy. The calendula is able to permeate through the granular layer and so repair the burned skin from very deep down.

Tagetes is more biased towards helping the respiratory tract. It helps with coughs and colds and mucous build up. It is also ant-parasitic so can be useful for intestinal worms but also candida too.

Recipes for Healthy Living – The medicine cupboard!!

Here are a few recipes which will help you to guard against natures cruelty! (x denotes how many drops in your mix e.g 1x lavender = I drop of lavender essential oil)

Tooth ache

Your grandmother would tell you to look for oil of cloves and she would be right. Clove essential oil is wonderful to help ease the pain until you can get yourself to the dentist.

1 x clove

1 x lavender

1 x yarrow

1 x spikenard

Blend into about 10 ml of vegetable and rub onto the side of your jaw.

Ear ache

These are nasty things and this should only be used as an emergency prevention before you visit the doctor. Ear infections can spread very fast so please do not rely on essential oils here.

3 x tea tree

1 x lavender

1 x Rosemary

Mix into 10 ml of slightly warmed carrier oil. Stroke into the side of the face and also along the jaw line. You may also want to put a small amount onto a cotton bud and place gently inside of the ear. Putting a warm flannel over the area helps the oils to get to work treating the infection and easing the pain quickly.

For epilepsy safety you can omit rosemary.

Tension Headache

2 x Lavender

1 x Basil

1x Rosemary

Mix into 10 mls of carrier oil and massage onto the temples and forehead. Massage into the muscles which go down either side of the spine in your neck. Work also into the sore points which run around the base of your skull.

For epilepsy safety you can replace rosemary with geranium oil.

Nausea and Sickness

1 x chamomile

1 x peppermint

1 x mandarin

1 x tea tree

1 x ginger

Mix into 10 ml of carrier oil or add to a warm bath. Rub either in a clockwise direction over the abdomen around the belly button, on the throat and chest, or onto the inside of the wrist. Go with what feels right for you. You will be able to feel where the symptoms are most affected. Placing the oils onto the inside of the arm helps to get the oils quickly into the system

(Not for use for morning sickness in pregnancy)

Diarrhoea

To treat the dreaded lurgy we use ginger which is wonderful for any condition where the body is struggling to cope with excess moisture.

2 x Ginger

1 x Coriander

2 x Tea tree

1 x Lavender

Mix into 10 ml of carrier oil and rub onto the abdomen in a clockwise direction circling the belly button.

Also rub 1 x tea tree onto the wrist every 20 minutes or as often as you remember.

Haemorrhoids

This painful condition is caused by the strangulation of a blood vessel so we use the circulatory qualities of geranium to reduce the effects.

2 x geranium in sitz bath, or 5 x geranium in a normal bath.

For bleeding haemorrhoids make a cold compress and place on the area for 5 minutes. Ensure you eat plenty of fibre and drink lots of water through the day to soften stools and allow the oils to do their work.

In addition

Add to a blank cream or lotion:

2 x lavender

2 x geranium

2 x myrrh

2 x roman camomile

Apply to the bottom at least three times daily until the symptoms are reduced.

Colds and 'Flu symptoms

It goes without saying there is a big difference between a cold and influenza. If it seems your symptoms are becoming worse after a couple of days please visit your doctor. Influenza kills - do not take chances.

I have broken the treatments down into symptoms. Feel free to whack them all in one preparation if you are really suffering.

Stuffy Nose Rub

1 x Lemon

1 x Eucalyptus

1 x Myrrh

1 x Tea tree

Mix into 10 ml of carrier oil or a cream or lotion. Rub across the forehead, around the temples and under the eyes on the cheek bones. The oils will have very quick access to the sinuses this way.

Alternatively add to a warm bath.

Lower Temperature

Fevers are nature's way of purging the body of infection. They are a healthy and useful thing. However in children in particular they can be unsettling, dangerous and uncomfortable. This makes a lovely respite from the heat.

1 x camomile

1 x geranium

1 x peppermint

1 x tea tree

Make a cold compress and place onto forehead or back of the neck.

Warming lotion

Just as we get the flushes, a cold can bring shivers too. This warming lotion smells like Christmas and feels like you are toasty by the fireside.

Add to 2oz bottle of blank lotion or carrier oil

1x ginger

1 x black pepper

1 x geranium

1 x orange

Rub into your joints and feet and you will start to feel your temperature steady itself.

Sore throat
Add:

2 x lavender

2 x tea tree to 2 fl oz warm water.

I also add ½ a tablet of aspirin too.

Gargle and spit, repeating until all of the preparation has been used.

Zap the Bug!

Mix into a 2 fl oz blank lotion. Use and when required. If you do not have all of the oils just use a selection off the list.

3 x tea tree

1 x lavender

1x elemi

1 x inula

2 x manuka

2x kanuka

1 x ravensara

Rub onto the inside of your wrist as often as you remember.

Recipes for Relaxation
(x denotes how many drops in your mix e.g 1x lavender = I drop of lavender essential oil)

It is impossible to list all the treatments for stress because there are as many different ones as people and situations. You will see there are number of oils which creep up over and over again, they will give you clues how to blend your own mixes.

Calming Evaporator Mix
2 x lavender

2 x camomile

2 x geranium

2 x ylang ylang

If you do not have an evaporator, use boiling water and place the bowl somewhere warm put mine on top of the wood burner.

Gentle Sleep
I have separated insomnia off for habitual non sleepers. This one is gorgeously relaxing and warming so you drift off as soon as your head hits the pillow. I would also suggest using two preparations together. You may want to do a bath then a lotion for instance, or even add the oils to an evaporator too.

2 x Lavender

2 x Camomile

1 x Geranium

1 x Sandalwood

1 x Frankincense

Add to a warm bath or evaporator. Blend into 2 fl oz body lotion to be applied 20 minutes before bead to the back of the neck and shoulders as well as the inside of the arm.

Insomnia Lotion

2 x lavender

3 x marjoram

Blend into a 2 fl oz body lotion and use first about an hour before bed and repeat every 20 minutes until you drift off. This treatment works on the central nervous system to reprogram your mind to go to sleep. You may find you need to use it for up to a week before your body stars to respond quickly to the treatment.

Aching Joints Massage Oil

2 x lavender

2 x juniper

1 x black pepper

1 x rosemary

1 x frankincense

Mix into 1 fl oz of vegetable oil or simply add neat essential oils add to your bath.

Massage into the most painful parts, remembering that the oils are able to flush there themselves too. This should help if there are parts you cannot reach on your back for instance, rub as close the area as you can get.

Sensuous Massage Oil

Stress can take its own tolls on a loving relationship. This makes a really special way to reconnect.

2 x ylang ylang

2 x sandalwood

2 x jasmine

1 x geranium

1 x nutmeg

Add into 2 fl ozs of a thick vegetable carrier oil such as almond (be aware of nut allergies) or jasmine oil.

Stroke liberally all over the body using long flowing strokes.

Worry Treatment

1 x Lavender

1 x Geranium

1 x Rose

1 x Frankincense

1 x Violet Resinoid

Use anyway which feels right. Add to 2 fl ozs of massage oil, or to your bath. You may also want to make an evaporator oil or even a candle to have burning in the background to calm you.

Recipes for Skin Care, Body and Beauty

(x denotes how many drops in your mix e.g 1x lavender = I drop of lavender essential oil)

Facial Cleansing Lotions

Purchase a very basic skin cleansing lotion for your local beauty store. Then add in essential oils as follows:

Dry skin:

2 x Geranium

2 x ylang ylang

1 x carrot seed oil

1 x cypress oil

Oily or spotty skin:

2 x lavender

1 x tea tree

1 x oakmoss resin

1 x grapefruit

Smoker's skin

1 x frankincense

1 x neroli

2 carrot

1 x oakmoss resin

Nourishing cream

This lusciously thick cream makes a delicious emollient for your skin. Treat your face using it as a night cream or copy my trick and use it under your make up for a gorgeously silky smooth finish for your make up.

1/4 cup coconut oil

1/8 cup shea butter

1/8 cup cocoa butter

1 Tbsp aloe vera juice

1 Tbsp carrier oil

5-10 drops essential oils

Method:

Heat the shea butter, the coconut oil, and cocoa butter in a saucepan over a low heat until it is completely melted.

Remove it from the heat and then add in the aloe vera juice, your carrier and essential oils. Give it a really good stir to ensure they are all very well combined.

Pour into your jar and allow it to thicken.

Do not put the top on until it is completely cooled and set. This prevents any moulds from forming.

Essential oils choices:

Dry & normal skins
2 x rose

2 x geranium

1 x frankincense

1 x sandalwood

Greasy skins
2 x lavender

2 x ylang ylang

1 x tea tree

Hand and Nail Treatment
2 x tagetes

2 x myrrh

1 x sandalwood

1 x galbanum

3 x rose

3 x geranium

Body Lotion

It is very simple to get a blank lotion base from your local chemist, but for those who feel ambitious….

> 1 tablespoon beeswax
>
> 1 tablespoon petroleum jelly
>
> 2 tablespoons distilled water (have more ready in case you want to mix to a lighter cream)
>
> ½ cup of carrier oil
>
> 6 drops of your essential oils.

Combine your carrier oil, beeswax and petroleum jelly in a microwave safe container.

Heat the mixture on a medium temperature. Checking every thirty seconds until the ingredients are completely melted together.

Pour distilled water into the blend. Add the water very slowly. I like to do this in a food processor on the slowest setting but you can use a fork or a whisk. The more air you blend into the concoction the lighter and fluffier it will be. If you want a very runny lotion that is easy to apply and absorb simply add a little more water.

Stir in your chosen essential oils.

As the lotion cools you find that it thickens up too. Pour into your jar or bottle of choice.

It is possible to make a large batch of blank lotion and then simply add essential oils into cold lotions as and when you need them too. Remember these also make perfect carriers for your more medicinal blends as well as your beauty ones.

Luxury Nourishing Body Lotion

2 x rose

1 x jasmine

1 x sandalwood

1 x cardamom

Itching Skin
1 x lavender

2 x camomile maroc

Apply to affected area as and when required

Sunburn and after sun lotion
1 x lavender

3 x camomile

2 x peppermint

2 x cardamom

1 x patchouli

1 x sandalwood

Stroke on very gently!

After Sport Muscle Rub
1 x lavender

1 x juniper

1 x frankincense

1 x black Pepper

Apply to the limbs after showering to really make the muscles work to flush out toxins and tone up.

Cellulite Lotion
This blend has many diuretic properties to flush the toxins out of the body. Ensure you drink plenty of water when you use this preparation.

1 x grapefruit

1 x cypress

2 x fennel

2 x juniper

1 x black pepper

Rub into the skin working from the feet in upward strokes towards the pelvis. This helps the toxins to empty into the lymphatic system and drain away more easily.

These also work very well mixed into massage oil.

Scrubs

Did you know that your skin is actually made up from three different layers and that the cells on the top one are all dead? They naturally shed (which is what forms most of the dust in our houses!) to let new cells come through. Exfoliation is the correct term for taking off the top layer and this is one of the single best things you can do to get a younger looking glowing complexion.

Sugar Scrub

1 cup sugar or other granulated sweetener

1 cup carrier oil

Essential oils:

2 x geranium 2 x sandalwood

Blend all the ingredients together and then seal in an airtight container.

Facial Scrub

2 tablespoons wheat germ (ask at your health food store)

1 teaspoon honey

½ teaspoon of dried flower petals (eg roses, lavender, calendula, geranium petals)

Essential oils:

1 x rose

1 x sandalwood

1 x cardamom

1 x carrot seed

Mix together and smear across your face,

Massage in circular motions for gently exfoliate dead skin cells and expose fresh younger looking ones below

Wash away by splashing with warm water.

Watery Delights and Bathroom Pleasures

Hair Care

Conditioning Hot Oil Mask
2 oz Carrier oil

1 x patchouli

1 x jasmine

1 x geranium

1 x sandalwood

Warm the mix until it is hot but comfortable to have on your head. Smooth all through your hair. Make your hands into rigid spiders and with your fingers exert pressure on your scalp and massage in.

Your scalp should actually move quite a lot but the more stressed we are the tighter it becomes. Work at unlocking the tension and loosening your head.

Then wrap your head in a warm towl and languish, relaxing for 20 minutes.

Shampoo out.

Hair Rinses
These rinses are ancient recipes which not only make your scalp tingle but get the very shiniest gloss to your hair.

To a jug of warm water add a tea spoon of cider vinegar and

Dark hair – Rosemary x 2

Mousey and red hair – Camomile x 2

Blonde hair – Lemon x 1 and also the squeeze of a fresh lemon too.

Put the plug in the sink and repeatedly rinse through the hair until squeaky clean.

Bath Salts

These make wonderful gifts. Store them in pretty glass jars so that the colors can be seen. I like to layer different colors in the jar to co-ordinate with my friends bathrooms.

11b Dead Sea Salts

10 drops of essential oils

2 drops Food colouring (optional)

Mix together well so the color and the scents are all well combined. Decant into jars and put the top on immediately to guard against the salts getting wet.

Milk Bath

4 oz Dried Milk

½ oz of dried flower petals

6 drops of essential oils.

6 Circles of fabric 8 ins diameter

6 x Ribbons 6 ins long

Put the petals and the oils into a bag and shake so the oils are absorbed into the petals. Leave overnight. Then mix in the dried milk powder.

Place in the centre of the circle and then bunch up so it is confined and then secure with the ribbon.

Tie onto the bath taps as the water fills your bath for the real Cleopatra experience. (I am afraid this is the closest I could get to the ass's milk that she was reputed to have used!)

Bath Oils & Shower Gels

Naturally oils will float on the water, but it is possible to buy a product called sodium laureth sulphate which is what would make the oils disperse. I find it easier to buy a basic bubble bath and add oils or even just make a massage oil and mix it with a bit of liquid soap (you know the hand washes you can buy?) which does the same thing.

The same applies to shower gels. Simply pour out the contents of your bottle into a jug, mix in some essential oils and return to the container.

Be aware though, these added chemicals can be more irritating to sensitive skins.

4 fl oz Carrier Oil

1 tablespoon of liquid soap (optional)

5-10 drops essential oils

Decant in a bottle for a lovely gift. Use 2 capfuls of the solution under the tap

Talc

One of the oddest things I find this day and age is talcum powder is now it is made without talc…what is it now then? I'm sure I don't know! Anyway it makes a wonderful end to a luxury bathing regime and you can make your own special blend of oils to go into them.

Just as lovely though, are single note talcs, that is just one oil in them. Make rose or lavender talcs for example.

Add 3 to 6 drops of essential oil to 4oz of talc-free powder. Put into a plastic container with a top on and shake it very, very, very hard! Consider that the powder will absorb the oils and then cake together so you are searching to smash those lumps to smithereens.

Leave for 3 weeks to let the oils completely permeate before use.

Essential Oil Bath Blends

Relaxing
2 x Lavender

1 x Camomile

2 x Geranium

1 x Patchouli

Sleep
2 x Lavender

1 x Valerian

1 x Camomile

1 x Marjoram

Sensuous
2 x Sandalwood

1 x ylang ylang

1 x nutmeg

1 x jasmine

Invigorating
This one works better for shower gels than bath oils.

1 x Melissa

1 x Rosemary

1 x Grapefruit

For patients with epilepsy replace rosemary with peppermint.

Aching Muscles
2 x lavender

2 x juniper

2 x frankincense

2 x geranium

Period Pain
2 x geranium

1 x camomile

1 x ylang ylang

1 x patchouli

1 x yarrow

Should of course, be administered with a large glass of red wine and three bars of chocolate!!!

Uplifting
2 x melissa

1 x geranium

2 x bergamot

1 x myrrh

Aromatherapy In Your Home
In addition to the lovely fragrance your home takes on you can keep it far more hygienic too. Many of these recipes are very ancient, some of them medieval, from a time where herbs were the only way to heal one's body. They are romantic, whimsical and will transport you back to simpler days.

Microwave Cleaner
Bowl of boiling water

3 x lemon oil

Place into the microwave and turn it on full blast for two minutes.

Wipe clean with a damp cloth. The greasy stains come off easily and the lemon oil disinfects and re-scents the oven.

Antibacterial Spray
I use this for wiping down all the surfaces if we have a bug in the house, but you could use it for cleaning kitchen surfaces too. (It does however flavour foods which touch it which is why I don't use it all the time!) The vodka helps to dissolve the essential oils.

4 fl oz distilled water

1 teaspoon vodka

2 x lemon

2 x tea tea

2 x manuka

2 x kanuka

Mix well and then decant into a spray bottle

Candles

The easiest candles are made from a sheet of beeswax (craft stores or Ebay) and a piece of string wick.

A sheet will make four small candles.

Cut it in half vertically, and then cut each half into half again across the diagonal. This will mean you have four triangles.

Lay your wick alongside the longest edge of the triangle, and smear oil in a line alongside the string.

It is important to ensure you do not put the oil on the string as it smells very bitter when the oils burn. This way they simply evaporate as the beeswax melts.

Christmas Cheer
2 x orange

2 x cinnamon

1 x nutmeg

1 x clove

Romance
1 x jasmine

1 x sandalwood

1 x ylang ylang

Room sprays

Whether you want a party vibe, a sultry sensation or some Christmas cheer use your oils in room sprays and evaporators to change the scent and atmosphere in a room.

4 fl oz distilled water

1 teaspoon vodka

Party Vibe

2 x mandarin

2 x melissa

1 x bergamot

1 x myrrh

Restful

2 x lavender

2 x camomile

1 x patchouli

1 x sandalwood

Wardrobe and Drawer Sachets

Soak lavender seeds with 2 drops of lavender oil and one of cedar wood oil. Pour the seeds into fabric sachets or bags to scent linen and keep away the moths!

Sleep Pillows

These sachets are actually inserts that are either slipped into, or can be sewn into pillows and removed for washing.

2 cups lavender seeds

½ cup dried hop flowers

½ camomile dried flower heads

6 x lavender

2 x valerian

2 x 8 ins squares of muslin

Blend together and shake well to ensure all the flowers are coated with essential oils.

Meanwhile stitch together the two pieces of muslin. Complete three sides and turn the pocket inside out. Fill with the flowers and then finish stitching the final side.

Slot inside your pillowcase for restful sleep

Scented Ink
Now, here is witchery in its very best form. Imbue your love letters, checks and even your Christmas cards with a magical air of mystery all of your own.

Using just one oil works best so you can have a single note of rose, jasmine, geranium or my favourite beguiling scent…ylang ylang

¼ teaspoon vodka

3 drops essential oil

Bottle of ink

Carefully stir in the essence and alcohol into the ink.

Aromatherapy in the garden
Aromatherapy has very few uses in the garden as the wide open spaces mean the oils dissipate into the air too quickly to have many effects. Animals and insects however, are used to sniffing out weak scents and so the majority of uses work best for them.

Shoo Fly!
There is nothing worse than spending an age preparing a lovely picnic for your garden party then being marauded by wasps and mozzies all afternoon.

3 x Citronella into a bowl of warm water or in a candle.

Get out, you dirty dawg!
This is an ancient aboriginal remedy.

Smear eucalyptus oil over your gate posts and along your perimeter to deter dogs from your property.

Bee welcome
Beekeepers use lemongrass oil to attract swarms of bees into their hives. Just a couple of drops here and there around the garden will have it humming in no time and then just watch your flowers bloom.

Aromatherapy For The Mind
Did you know with all the amazing things we can do with a computer scientists are still nowhere near being able to create one which can process information and manage as many operations as the human brain? With so many things going on inside of our heads is no wonder that sometimes we find it harder to manage our thoughts effectively sometime.

By now you should have a handle on how to mix oils and ways you can administer them for yourself so here are some ideas of oils to use to direct your thoughts. Use them to blend into your preparations.

Exam Focus
Rosewood or Ho wood

Meditation and Prayer
Frankincense, myrrh, angelica, olibanum

Creativity
Basil, bergamot, jasmine

Grief
Rose

Confidence
Frankincense, labdanum, melissa, bergamot

Anxiety

Rose, valerian, bergamot, camomile, frankincense, marjoram

Trauma

Rose, camphor (but no more than one drop and not suitable in **epilepsy or pregnancy)**

Safety Advice

Essential oils are not suitable for everyone. The way they encourage the hormones in the systems to alter can create damaging effects in some groups.

The main people to have concerns are:

1. Diabetes sufferers
2. Epilepsy patients
3. Pregnant women
4. Breast feeding women

Diabetes

People with diabetes can safely use most essential oils with the exception of angelica oil. Oils which encourage the pancreas to work more effectively are dill and fennel and as such these are very helpful to suffers.

Epilepsy

Some essential oils are what is called neuro-toxic which makes them dangerous not only to suffers of epilepsy but also some types of schizophrenia too. Essential oils to avoid are: Rosemary, fennel, sage, eucalyptus, hyssop, camphor and spike lavender (Lavendula latifolia)

Pregnant Women

There are many actions which can make essential oils dangerous in pregnancy. All essential oils should be avoided during the first 16 weeks then you should avoid Angelica, Black Pepper, Clove, Cypress, Eucalyptus, Ginger, Helichrysum, Marjoram, Myrrh, Nutmeg, Oregano, Peppermint, Roman Chamomile, Basil, Cassia, Cinnamon bark, Clary Sage, Lemongrass, Rosemary, Thyme, Vetiver, Wintergreen, White Fir

Essential oils can be tasted in breast milk and so you may find it puts baby off feeding. Whilst Carrot Seed Oil will enhance milk flow, geranium help sooth engorged breasts and Marigold can heal cracked nipples all others should be used with care.

If baby does stop feeding stop using oils for a day and see what happens.

Chemotypes

Just as there are many different looking lavender plants so they all produce slightly different oils. You can see the different chemotypes in their latin names. Some chemotypes of an essential oil can render it dangerous for use Lavendula stoechas for instance is very dangerous in pregnancy, and latifolia can induce fits. Always read the label carefully.

Conclusion

Well, if you have found your way this far through the book, I'll take it as a compliment! I hope that you have found it useful and perhaps I may even have been able to ignite just a tiny spark of interest within you.

I hope so, because like all those generations of healers who have gone before me, I feel it is my responsibility to Mother Earth to help pass on that knowledge to healers yet to come. I would love to think you may be one of those too.

As you wander off into the sunset with your precious little collection of nature's juices, let me share with you a quote from the wonderful poet John Keats. He said:

"The poetry of the earth is never dead"

How wonderfully true. Just as my knowledge has been passed to you of the flowers we have on our planet now, then nature will hybridise and evolve new plants for the diseases of our children's children. This has always been its way.

If, for no other reason than that (and yes, there are myriad more) we must protect our planet and preserve nature's bounty for the generations who follow in our shadows.

Our social conscience has snaked around and taken a U-turn. More readily, we hear the whispers of the ancient peoples who still dwell so closely with their lands; the tribesmen, the aboriginals, the Native American Indians, and their peers. It is time to heed to their warnings and join together to ensure these medicines continue to have habitats in which to grow. For not only do our physical selves need healing but these glorious pastures give you hearts a chance to grow quiet and soar. So important to our healthy souls.

Chief Luther Standing Bear will conclude far better than I ever could.

"Wherever forests have not been mowed down, wherever the animal is recessed in their quiet protection, wherever the earth is not bereft of four-footed life - that to the white man is an 'unbroken wilderness.'

But for us there was no wilderness, nature was not dangerous but hospitable, not forbidding but friendly. Our faith sought the harmony of man with his surroundings; the other sought the dominance of surroundings.

For us, the world was full of beauty; for the other, it was a place to be endured until he went to another world.

But we were wise. We knew that man's heart, away from nature, becomes hard."

Glossary

Antifungal – Fighting fungal infections such as athletes foot or candida

Antiviral – Guarding against viruses such as E coli and influenza

Benzene – Colorless liquid which is a set of hydrocarbons used in extraction

Carcinogenic – Creating cancerous cells

Cephalic – Relating to the brain

Chemotypes – Differing species of the same plant

CO_2 Extraction – Process of using carbon dioxide as a means of separating essential oils from their original plant matter

Cohabition – A process of fractional distillation where missing parts of an oil are replaced to make it complete

Concrete – A solvent used for extraction of essential oils

Contraindication – Providing danger; reasons why a process should not be used

Diabetes – Disease derived from problems relating to blood sugar and insulin production

Digestive – Bodily process where the body takes energy and nutrients from food and the processes bodily waste

Diuretic – Increasing the need for urination

Enzymes Proteins able to bring about changes in the body

Epilepsy – Illness involving seizures and vacant episodes

Extraction – Process of removing essential oils from their plant matter

Fractional Distillation – Process of extraction where steam is used to purge oil from plant matter

Haemorrhoids – Painful rectal condition of constricted blood vessels

Haemorrhagic – Increasing blood loss ie causing haemorrhage

Hexane –colorless liquid used in extraction of essential oils

Hybridise – cross breed

Limbic system – part of the brain concerned with learning, memory, emotions and spatial awareness

Misnomer – Incorrect name

Olfactory – pertaining to smell

Osmosis – Diffusion of fluid through a membrane

Permeable – Something which can be penetrated or passed through

Respiratory – pertaining to breathing in the body

Full Disclaimer

by SEQ Legal

(1)   Introduction

This disclaimer governs the use of this ebook. [By using this ebook, you accept this disclaimer in full. / We will ask you to agree to this disclaimer before you can access the ebook.]

(2)   Credit

This disclaimer was created using an SEQ Legal template.

(3)   No advice

The ebook contains information about aromatherapy and the use of essential oils. The information is not advice, and should not be treated as such.

[You must not rely on the information in the ebook as an alternative to qualified medical advice from a health professional. advice from an appropriately qualified professional. If you have any specific questions about any medical matter you should consult an appropriately qualified professional.]

[If you think you may be suffering from any medical condition you should seek immediate medical attention. You should never delay seeking medical advice, disregard medical advice, or discontinue medical treatment because of information in the ebook.]

(4)   No representations or warranties

To the maximum extent permitted by applicable law and subject to section 6 below, we exclude all representations, warranties, undertakings and guarantees relating to the ebook.
Without prejudice to the generality of the foregoing paragraph, we do not represent, warrant, undertake or guarantee:

> that the information in the ebook is correct, accurate, complete or non-misleading;

> that the use of the guidance in the ebook will lead to any particular outcome or result; or

in particular, that by using the guidance in the ebook you will heal disease or work in any way as a cure for illness.

(5) Limitations and exclusions of liability

The limitations and exclusions of liability set out in this section and elsewhere in this disclaimer: are subject to section 6 below; and govern all liabilities arising under the disclaimer or in relation to the ebook, including liabilities arising in contract, in tort (including negligence) and for breach of statutory duty.

We will not be liable to you in respect of any losses arising out of any event or events beyond our reasonable control.

We will not be liable to you in respect of any business losses, including without limitation loss of or damage to profits, income, revenue, use, production, anticipated savings, business, contracts, commercial opportunities or goodwill.

We will not be liable to you in respect of any loss or corruption of any data, database or software.

We will not be liable to you in respect of any special, indirect or consequential loss or damage.

(6) Exceptions

Nothing in this disclaimer shall: limit or exclude our liability for death or personal injury resulting from negligence; limit or exclude our liability for fraud or fraudulent misrepresentation; limit any of our liabilities in any way that is not permitted under applicable law; or exclude any of our liabilities that may not be excluded under applicable law.

(7) Severability

If a section of this disclaimer is determined by any court or other competent authority to be unlawful and/or unenforceable, the other sections of this disclaimer continue in effect.

If any unlawful and/or unenforceable section would be lawful or enforceable if part of it were deleted, that part will be deemed to be deleted, and the rest of the section will continue in effect.

(8) Law and jurisdiction

This disclaimer will be governed by and construed in accordance with English law, and any disputes relating to this disclaimer will be subject to the exclusive jurisdiction of the courts of England and Wales.